Fifty Shades
of
Oral Pleasure

A BEDSIDE GUIDE TO GOING
DOWN FOR HIM AND HER

MARISA BENNETT

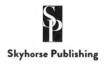

Skyhorse Publishing

A special thank you to my friends at Ravenous Romance for providing the inspiring erotica excerpts!

Skyhorse Publishing books may be purchased in bulk at special discounts for sales promotion, corporate gifts, fund-raising, or educational purposes. Special editions can also be created to specifications. For details, contact the Special Sales Department, Skyhorse Publishing, 307 West 36th Street, 11th Floor, New York, NY 10018 or info@skyhorsepublishing.com.

Skyhorse® and Skyhorse Publishing® are registered trademarks of Skyhorse Publishing, Inc.®, a Delaware corporation.

Visit our website at www.skyhorsepublishing.com.

10 9 8 7 6 5 4 3

Library of Congress Cataloging-in-Publication Data is available on file.

ISBN: 978-1-62636-089-1

Printed in the United States of America

DEDICATION

To Patrick and Eddie.
You're welcome.

CONTENTS

INTRODUCTION

T here is a sexual revolution upon us. With even the most taboo of erotica novels hitting the mainstream, the idea that "sex sells" has transformed from an old advertising mantra into a new, sometimes-dressed-up-in-leather, universal embrace of the things we do behind closed doors. Luckily for us, this includes one of the very best kinds of copulation: mind-blowing oral sex.

While some Puritanical facets of society would like to say that oral sex is a dirty invention of the porn industry or the sexually deviant media, going down has been around for as long as the owners of penises and vaginas have used their mouths to kiss. Even in the ancient city of Pompeii, known for its volcanic demise, archaeologists have found frescoes and other forms of artwork depicting oral sex. Historians are divided as to its purpose: because of the artwork's placement in the baths, some think it's an advertisement for sexual services offered, while others think it was just a funny picture used to help patrons remember where they left their clothes. Even in ancient China, there are paintings of Empress Wu Zetian of the T'ang Dynasty receiving cunnilingus from her noblemen. (It's been debated whether these images were accurate depictions, or just the ancient likeness to a modern political cartoon. Whichever the case, I say rock on Empress.)

From past to present, ancient to modern, analog to digital, oral sex has been and is a passionate expression of human sexuality that makes having a mouth and an erogenous zone feel like one of the seven wonders of the world. If anything, consider this book to be tipping its hat to the history of head-givers past! This is an enthusiastic guide to His and Her oral trysts, from basic anatomy, grooming trends, orgasmic techniques every couple should master, to thrilling oral sex positions with artful sketches to guide you. I've even included a few *inspirational* sexy stories to get your blood pumping. Now, you were given a mouth for more than just the purposes of speaking and eating cotton candy. Read on and get using it!

Part One

Her

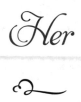

"It was love at first sight, at last sight, at ever and ever sight."

—Vladimir Nabokov,
Lolita

"I want to do
with you what spring
does with the
cherry trees."

—Pablo Neruda

INTRODUCTION TO PLEASURING HER ORALLY

⌒

Penetrative sex is a crapshoot for women. Studies show that only 25 percent of women regularly orgasm from penetration, which means that a majority of ladies are putting out and not getting much in return. At least, not from p-in-the-v sex. But with oral, it's different: the focus is on her, and she's much more likely to get off. Women's orgasms are amazing: where male orgasms tend to last 6 seconds, an average female orgasm lasts 20 seconds, and most women can have multiple orgasms in a single romp! Going down, eating out, cunnilingus, whatever you call it, oral sex is an intimate experience: you're face to face with a part of her very few people get to be intimately acquainted with.

WHAT'S UP DOWN THERE: A GUIDE TO LADYBITS ANATOMY

⌒

Before you get down, you should take a look at where you're going. Whether you're a native of vagina-land or a backpacking visitor (Or even a new tourist! Welcome!), it's worth it to take a look at the map. While we normally use the word "vagina" to talk about the whole ladybits ecosystem, technically "vagina" only refers to the vaginal opening. Serious misnomer, since the vagina is such a small part of a woman's whole sexual experience: while it may be the star of the show in penetrative sex, if you want to really please a woman you don't need to go deeper, you want to spread out! The word "vagina" comes from the Latin word for sheath—you know, the place where you put your sword. But anyone with a good sword-holder between her legs can tell you there's more to going down there than just the female end of an electrical socket.

The right term for the kit and caboodle is "vulva," a vaguely foreign word (try it with a Russian accent) that has potential for sexiness, although since it's not often used colloquially it still has the ring of a medical term. Women's vulvas are very different, which can create plenty of insecurity for anyone who doesn't look quite like the diagram in her health class textbook. Like snowflakes, no two pussies are exactly the same, but they all share the same basic parts that you should get to know.

LABIA MAJORA
(THE OUTER PUSSY LIPS)

I love the neat organization of the vulva, almost like someone has sorted the ladybits into charming little pink folders for easy access. The outermost "folder" is called the *labia majora,* literally the "big lips." The outer skin varies in sensitivity, but it can often be more receptive than you would think, when you consider how many women have their outer labia doused in wax and the hair ripped out!

The outer labia are physiologically similar to the scrotum, but don't expect it to be as delicate as a set of balls: your mileage may vary, but many women enjoy having their lips stroked, massaged, kissed, rubbed and otherwise played with during pussy play. As always be gentle and follow her lead!

LABIA MINORA
(THE INNER PUSSY LIPS)

The inner folder, tucked neatly inside the outer lips, is called the *labia minora.* These folds are softer and more sensitive than her outer lips: they are sometimes called "nymphae," which I think is just lovely. The labia minora can look quite different from one woman to another, with some bigger or smaller, and varying in coloring. The inner lips also change in appearance when the woman is aroused, usually becoming larger and either darker or brighter (think "rosier") in color as blood rushes to the area. Because these inner lips are more sensitive than the outer lips, your attentions will likely be rewarded if you gently lick, suck, and kiss all around here, paying attention to her responses. One good move is to slowly trace a line from her vagina up to the spot just below her clit, moving your tongue (or your wet or lubed finger) between her pussy lips, parting them as you go. This is a nice teasing move that helps you gauge her response. Does she try to move you faster? Push you up toward her clit? Sigh and lie back to enjoy what you're doing? Pay attention and follow her lead to give her the most pleasure!

CLITORIS

The love button. The little man in the boat. The mysterious clit, only revealed to the most astute and attentive lover—well, let's hope not, because if she wants to come, then you should be intimately acquainted with her clitoris.

First, an introduction: The clitoris is a mass of nerve endings set right above the vagina, neatly tucked beneath where the left and right lips of the labia minora meet up, under a fold of skin called the clitoral hood.

Its only obvious purpose is to stimulate pleasure; a fantastic fact, especially considering that a woman's orgasm is not necessary for conception, making her pleasure evolutionarily unimportant. The clitoris has eight thousand nerve endings, double the number in the penis, all bundled up together. But the clit you see is just the tip of the iceberg. The visible clitoris is called the *glans clitoris* (like the glans or head of a penis), and it is the head of a larger system that branches out and down toward the vagina. This theory accounts for the sometimes-elusive g-spot, thought to be part of this network of nerves.

So the little clit is not to be ignored. But as Monty Python opined, "Why not start her off with a nice kiss? You don't have to go leaping straight for the clitoris like a bull at a gate." Aside from the fact that no one should be approaching the clitoris in any way that is bull-like, the point is that her clitoris is not an "on switch," and if you keep flicking it like that you're going to get punched in the face.

Even if a woman loves it when you rub her clit, your best bet is to start out with indirect stimulation and save rougher, more direct stimulation for when she's close to climax. There are plenty of ways for you to do this: licking and fondling her inner lips, working your way toward her clit. You can gently pull and tug on her pussy to make her clit rub up against the hood. You can even lick and fondle the hood itself for a closer indirect hit.

Once all systems are go and she's deep in a groove, you should switch it up a lot to see what seems to turn her on the most. But once she's indicated (through moans, screams, or by direct physical signs like pulling your hair or pushing you into her crotch) that you've gotten it *just right, that's it, right there*, then do a girl a favor and keep doing exactly what you're doing until she comes!

VAGINA

Vaginas are amazing, flexible, versatile things. They can stretch and squeeze to accommodate anything from a baby to a penis to a dildo, even an entire fist, if you're into that. And only with lube. Since there are fewer supersensitive nerve endings in and around the vagina than there are up by the clitoris, you don't want to focus all of your attentions there. Approach with caution the idea of "tongue-fucking" her: that move may be sexier in theory than actual practice, although your mileage may vary. Still, try adding a few fingers while you're focusing on her more sensitive spots, and she's in for a ride!

G-SPOT

When you're adding a few fingers, you should aim them in the direction of the g-spot, on the front wall of the vagina. This spot was named for Ernst Gräfenberg, and researchers have been studying and arguing about it since the 1600s. They're still arguing about it today: in 2009, British researchers conducting a questionnaire survey concluded that the g-spot did not exist, but more recent French experiments taking ultrasounds of women having sex have shown good evidence that the sensitive area exists, and changes while she's having sex. If you can't find it, don't be too concerned; just like any other move, this one works for some and not for others. But if you're exploring, try stroking the inside of her vagina, on the front wall about two inches in. Feel for an area with a rougher texture, and when you find it apply gentle pressure as you stroke. You can do this with the patented "come hither" wiggle, or make up your own technique!

GROOMING GUIDE FOR HER

It's just good manners to make sure that you're clean and tidy if you're going to be getting down. But that doesn't require any hair removal, it only means that you need to wash regularly, and maybe give your girl-fro a little shampoo and conditioner every now and again.

Removing your pubic hair is a style choice, not a health decision, and if you like rocking an untouched, (not so) virgin thicket between your legs, rock on. There are always people trying to tell women that we're gross for one reason or another, so just tell them to fuck off.

That's not to say that women who prune their bushes are all patsies in a big social scheme or anything. In fact, many women are choosing to groom their ladybits because they *want* to (SHOCK) and because they like it. I like how it looks, and I like how it feels! But there are varying degrees of grooming between natural and completely bushwhacked, you just have to find which works for you!

JUST A TRIM

GOOD NEWS! This technique is all win. Get yourself a nice trimmer from the drugstore; the ones made for bikini grooming are the best, but if you're shy, there are plenty of nondescript clippers. Set the clippers to a tidy length and go to town. You'll have less undergrowth to wade through, but you won't have to deal with ingrown hairs or newly grown stubble. You'll have to trim often to keep it maintained, so keep your trimmer charged!

SHAVING

Shaving is a cheap and easy way to get rid of your pubic hair. You probably already have the tools in your shower, and you know how to wield them. If you're just looking to keep your bikini line tidy and not to go completely bare, you just add that to your weekly rotation along with your underarm and leg shaving. Avoid painful razor burn by taking special care of your sensitive lady parts: take your time in the shower to get the area completely wet, and use plenty of shaving cream or gel. You can find bikini-specific shave cream that works especially well. Always use a nice razor, and follow up with a soothing lotion. You'll likely still get some redness and bumps, but they should calm down within a day or so. But by then it may be time for another shave.

WAX OFF

Shaving can be quick and easy, but it has lots of downsides as a consistent hair removal method. You have to shave almost every day, and the ingrown hairs ruin the "smooth and silky" look.

If you are sick of shaving and want your removal methods to last longer, you'll want to try waxing. The thought of letting someone pour hot melted wax down below the belt and then ripping it off is quite alarming, but honestly and sincerely—it's not that bad.

I've tried home waxing a few times with mixed results. There are a few different types of home wax-es, and I tried most of them in my quest to rid my-self of my own thick tangle without showing off my hoo-ha to some salon tech. But more on that later. If you're waxing at home, it's important to follow ALL

OF THE INSTRUCTIONS SO YOU DON'T BURN OR OTHERWISE MAIM YOUR PUSSY. You might also need to be very flexible, or have a very good friend (or sexy-times partner!) to help you with the hard-to-reach spots.

Strips: One type of wax comes pre-applied, sandwiched between cloth strips: I had to warm up the wax by rubbing them between my hands then peeling the strips apart. Then I placed it on my shorthairs, and quickly zipped it off in the direction that the hair grows. Since my hair is so thick, this technique was pretty useless for me, but if you have finer hair or you're just cleaning up the edges, these strips are so much less messy and so much easier to use than the tubs of wax.

Popsicle Stick: This kind of wax comes in a tub that you heat up in the microwave. Some of these also come with cloth strips to pull the wax off, but the one I like best works a little differently: you apply the melted wax with the popsicle stick, then wait for it to cool a little bit. Then you grab the corner of the wax and zip it off, pulling opposite to the direction that the hair grows.

Salon Waxing:

I had already abused my poor pubic hair with home waxing attempts when I decided to get a professional wax at a salon. I made the decision months earlier, but every time I thought to make an appointment all I could think of was how awkward it would be for a stranger to be interacting with my nether regions. But in the interest of good nonfiction, I made the appointment. I went to a local spa, where they set me up in a massage room on a soft, deep cushion. The technician was quick and professional, telling me about the process as she went through the motions. The room was dim except for a bright dentist-style light she had focused helpfully on my crotch. She put baby powder on my skin to keep the wax from sticking, then spread warm, seaweed-green wax right along my bikini line. It smelled good, kind of like beeswax. She pushed a strip of cloth down onto the wax and then before I had time to flinch it was gone, along with a big patch of hair. She shook on another layer of baby powder and applied gentle pressure to keep my skin from stinging, but it wasn't necessary, any pain I felt was momentary. After a few more quick zips I was finished. I've already made my appointment for next month!

Dying it (The Betty):

Getting rid of your hair is a matter of style— what if you want to go the other way and rock a stylish bush? One new trend is to dye it! Only about 50 percent of women have carpets that match their drapes, so dyeing the hair down there can be great for "blondes" who really want to be blondes, for aging women who would like to cover up some grays, or for women who just want to try out a new do. Use a dye made for pubic hair use, like the products from Betty Beauty, which has colors ranging from natural shades like brunettes, auburns, and blondes, to bright fun colors like pink, purple, blue and green. This could be even more fun with some creative grooming: you could use your trimmer to create a pink heart for Valentine's Day, a nice strip of green to celebrate spring; perhaps a bright blue lightning bolt just for fun!

ORAL SEXNIQUES TO TURN HER ON

The bad news is there is no super secret move that will turn all women into a melted puddle at your feet. All women are different, and a woman's tastes may change from romp to romp, so the best trick I can give you is to read your partner. Pay attention to all the signs she's giving you, from the words she's saying (and "oh, yeah" counts) to the way she's moving and breathing, to the touch and feel of her body. But everybody says that, and it doesn't give you anywhere to start. So I've put together some more tips that can help you explore her body and find out exactly how to make her say, "More, please!"

SAY THE ABCs

This trick is tried-and-true, and it will help you suss out how your partner likes to stroke it. Use your tongue to spell out the ABCs on her pussy. This is a good beginner technique because as you're twirling the letters, up, down, left, right, you can try to feel out which movements she likes best. Slow down and change your pressure while you move across her entire vulva, feeling out where she wants you. This is a good trick to have at the ready to help with "pussy calibration," but once you know what your lady likes, you should move on, since the ever-changing motions can get frustrating as she gets closer to coming.

HUM!

You don't want to seem bored, or strange, so don't just hum a little ditty to her pussy. Instead, incorporate some noises of enjoyment into your oral experience: with her clit in your mouth, or with your mouth pressed up against her pussy, make a little "mmmmmmm" noise to let her know you like what you're doing. The gentle vibrations can feel really good, and the primal, enthusiastic noises are a serious turn-on, especially when combined with so many other sensations!

PANTS OFF DANCE OFF

This tip is great for getting started. The rule is that she keeps her pants on until she's ready, moaning, and tearing them off herself. This way she's ready and begging for it before your mouth meanders south. Until then, use your whole hand to fondle and manipulate her pussy lips from the outside of her pants. Don't focus on her clit or try to pinpoint a specific spot to touch; this is more of a "macro pussy massage." Let her grind against you as you make out; it might seem old-school, but that just adds to its appeal.

Use your hands: lay your hand on her whole pussy, with your palm by her clit and your fingers resting on her pussy lips, then move your hand to pull back toward her belly button. This slides the clit in and out of its little "hood," essentially jerking her off. Try back and forth movements as well, right over her clitoris. Sitting either in front or behind her, put your whole hand over her pussy again, with your fingertips in line with her clit, then move your whole hand back and forth, kind of like an old-school DJ scratching a record. Try not to create too much friction: you don't want to rub the fabric of her pants against her clit, because without any lube that can be painful! By the time she tears her pants off, you won't have to do much more to get her off!

NOW KISS

Some like their cunnilingus with a side of romance, so pucker up when you go down. Kiss gently along the inside of her outer pussy lips, then circle inward, leaving soft kisses along her inner labia. Trace kisses from her vagina to her clitoris, quick and lightly at first, then slower with a bit more pressure. Switch to more passionate kissing: part your lips and gently suck on her pussy before you pull away. Start using your tongue like you would when kissing: rhythmically stroke her clit and inner labia, moving your tongue with your lips. Move in the same patterns you traced at the beginning, changing the speed and pressure. Focus your attentions on her clit, using the same gentle sucking, kissing move you used before. Follow her lead and let her tell you how she likes it. When she's ready to come, stay right where you are, keeping the pressure and speed steady—unless she's yelling "harder!" or "faster!", in which case, she's the boss!

ON THE BUTTON

But what do you do with the clit? All the advice says you're doing it wrong if you ignore the clit, but once it's looking you in the face, what do you do with it? Some women don't want you touching their clit at all, and some women only like it after you've gotten them warmed up. But if you know your lady loves to have her button pushed, you need to give it some extra attention. Here are some ways to stimulate that needy clit:

SWIRL IT

Draw circles around her clit with your tongue. Start wide, pausing to nibble on her lips as you slide by. Move toward the clit, making it the center of the concentric circles you're drawing across her vulva. Every other swoop, reverse the direction. Draw the circles tighter and tighter until you reach her clitoris, reversing direction and alternating your speed. Continue tracing circles around her clitoris, flicking your tongue over clit until she hits her groove.

BOP IT

Suck her clit into your mouth, holding it steady while you gently smack it about with your tongue. Come at it from all angles, batting it around. This will drive even the most hardy clitoris wild! Keep your suction gentle, just enough to keep her in place as you bop her clit. If she seems to respond to one bop more than others, add more of those into your rotation. Just don't keep smacking her the same way for too long, since it could desensitize her, and make it harder for her to come! But as she climbs toward climax, you should make your moves more regular and switch to a steady rhythm to help drum her home.

SUCK IT

You're not trying to give her a lower hickey, but don't be afraid to suck a little clit. Pop the clit into your mouth, then suck gently to draw it farther into your mouth. When you begin, suck as you would when you're kissing, alternating sucking with other soft fondling and massaging moves with your lips and tongue. Try giving the clit a mini "blow job," sucking on it while sliding it in and out of your mouth.

LICK IT

Ever heard of the term "flicking the bean"? Don't take it so literally. You'll notice none of these tips tell you to flick your tongue against her love button at the speed of light, because that move, while sadly quite popular, is shit. Your mouth is not a vibrator, and you're just going to wear yourself out, so just retire this move and write it on your list of "ways porn is wrong." Instead of flicking, you should concentrate on licking. Trace a slow line up between her pussy lips, right up to her clit. When your tongue hits that peak, roughly slide it up and over, then start again. Leave some time between strokes, and try not to confuse rough with "hard, unyielding tongue." Get animalistic and lap her up, but don't spend too much time slobbering on her. Alternate wide, wet strokes with more precise ones.

HANDS AND MOUTH

Many women find it easier to come when they have something to hold on to: in this case, you're going to want to add some penetration. You don't want to try to go too deep, since most of the more sensitive nerve endings are near the opening of the vagina. Use clean fingers to gently part her pussy lips, and keep doing what you're doing with your mouth as you move your fingers around—it may be interesting to stop and look, but you don't want to break your rhythm!

When you use your hands, try not to think about "penetrating" her in the traditional sense: your fingers are not a penis, and it's unlikely that simple in-

and-out movements will give her the kind of sensation she needs to get off. Instead, try a few different moves to see what she likes:

Small movements: Firstly, you may have better luck not moving much at all. Pussies are sensitive, and sometimes all she wants is something to hold on to while you're rocking her world. Start by gently inserting a finger into her vagina. Stroke inside of her gently while she gets used to your fingers. She may even grind against you or move so your fingers slide in and out. In this case, shift to make her motions easier, then continue what you're doing. Use your fingers to push against the insides of her pussy. Don't poke, and don't be too rough, just push gently. Pause and let her push back at you with her muscles, then you push again, gently. This back-and-forth can be really useful if your partner feels disconnected during oral sex—a concern that is common among some women.

G-Spot: This is a must-see location on your holiday down south! There really is no mystery to the g-spot: it's a bundle of nerve endings just inside the vagina (on the front wall, kind of like on the other side of her belly button) that many women like played with during sexy times. This erogenous zone is different for everyone, a clear illustration of the phrase "different strokes for different folks"! The g-spot is most likely part of a kind of "pleasure

system" made up of the clitoris and the other con-
nected nerve endings spread out around her vulva.
All the advice says to just stick in a finger and give a
little "come hither" wiggle, and this seems to work
for lots of people. If you're not having any luck, you
may have to spend some time spelunking. As you
stroke her g-spot, it swells and becomes more sensitive, so if you can't find the magic spot right away,
it could get easier as you play around. Contrary to
popular belief, though, the g-spot is not a magic bul-
let, it's just an added dimension of pleasure for her. I
like it best when the pressure on my g-spot is coun-
tered with pressure on my clit!

STEADY HAND

Cunnilingus shouldn't be all light fairy touches and
gentle strokes. Women vary widely in sensitivity, and
your partner may be more or less sensitive each time
you tango: if you head south and her legs snap shut,
she might be feeling too sensitive. You can still rock
her world: you just have to have a steady hand and a
quick tongue. Start with some massage foreplay: use
strong, consistent strokes, leaving your hands on her
body as long as possible as you rub her down. Remember that massage increases blood flow, so spend
more time around her breasts, her ass, and working
up her legs to her pussy—but leave that alone for a

bit. Wait for her to start responding to your handiwork before diving in, and when you do, keep your steady touch. Touch her with more of your hand: use your palm when you can, or where you'd usually use a fingertip, use the flat pads of your pointer and middle fingers. When you head to her clit, stroke it indirectly. Put your whole hand over her clit and rub in slow circles. Pause every now and then and just press gently, and let her grind against you. When you add oral, move in the same way: slowly, while letting her know where you're going to touch next. Keep your mouth on her for longer than necessary, and touch her deliberately. Let her move against you and follow her lead while keeping up your steady, strong strokes.

Kink for Her

Toys can add an extra level of fun to your oral sex session! Toys like tongue vibrators are made for oral experience, but you'll find that any of these toys can up the excitement. So break open your toy box—or stock up!

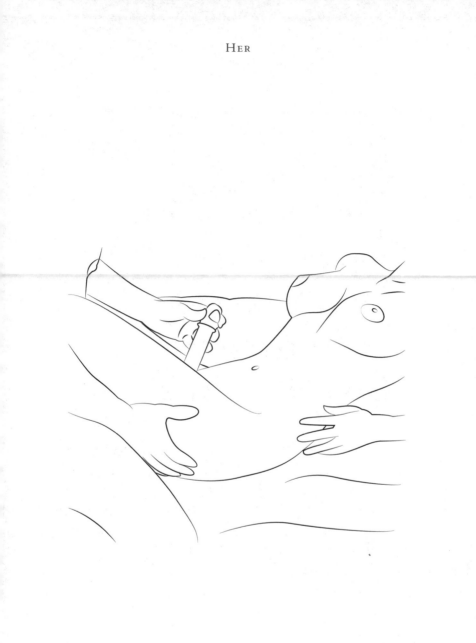

"She would lift her peignoir above her knees and say to her husband: "Give baby a kiss . . .""

—Isaac Babel,
First Love

Your rounded thighs are
like jewels,
the work of a master
hand.
You navel is a rounded bowl
that never lacks mixed wine.
Your belly is a heap of
wheat,
encircled with lilies.

Song of Solomon, 7:1-7:2

DILDO

Give a girl something to hold on to while you're blowing her mind! If your fingers are busy elsewhere, use her dildo! Get her sopping wet before you penetrate her, and move gently and slowly. Have her guide you while you put it in. Then, hold it in place while you go down on her, letting her move up and down on the toy. Or she can hold the dildo, and move it as she wants. How you do this will depend on your position, of course!

TONGUE VIBRATOR

The point of a vibrating tongue ring is to turn your mouth into her sex toy! Strap the contraption to your tongue and switch it on, then focus your attentions on her pussy. This is especially great if your partner needs a bit more stimulation to get off: it will save you time, and jaw pain!

The effectiveness of these depend on the quality of the product, since they have a tendency to slip off. You might find that the more expensive versions work better, but the truth is it's difficult to strap anything to your tongue. A more realistic alternative is to use a finger vibrator that straps to your finger, supercharging your touch! Alternate mouth moves with gentle strokes, and move it around to see where she likes it best!

WAND VIBRATOR

This is your standard vibe, and its name is quite appropriate. Wave your magic wand wherever you want on her body and watch the transformation. Get creative and use her personal massager to rub down her ass and thighs when you're getting her warmed up. If your tongue gets tired, let the wand fill in for you for a bit. Use it like the dildo: make sure she's wet then gently slide the wand into her.

REMOTE ACTIVATED VIBRATOR

Some vibrators can be activated remotely, either by an actual remote, or by something like the rhythm of the music you're playing! This kind of vibrator is very helpful in all kinds of sexual adventures, you just need to be creative! Play a quiz game with your partner, and "buzz" her when she gets an answer wrong! Hold on to the remote when you're having dinner together, and buzz her when she's taking a bite. She'll be begging for more before dessert!

A music-driven vibrator is great for foreplay and the main act! DJ her pussy by starting off slow, with some hot sexytime music, then set the playlist to get her off. If you time it right you'll have the music crescendoing as she does!

G-SPOT VIBRATOR

This vibe is made specifically to stroke her g-spot. If she craves deep stimulation while you're going down, you'll want to try one of these. They vary in appearance: some g-spot vibrators look like a long thin rod with an egg shaped bulb at the end, while others look more like a standard, phallus-shaped vibrator with an extra hook or bend at the end. Since women stimulate their g-spot in different ways, there are lots of different types to suit your needs! Read product descriptions and reviews to get a better idea before you purchase your new toy.

ANAL TOYS

If you're both down for butt stuff, oral can be a fun time to add in some anal play toys! Standard rules apply: if it goes in someone's butt, it goes nowhere else until it it disinfected, or you're gonna have a bad time. If you're planning to use different toys in one session, or if you're especially worried about contamination, invest in some female condoms. They're designed to stay in, and they won't slip in if you're being gentle enough!

BUTT PLUG

This thing is exactly what it sounds like. A small size is perfect for a beginner, but if you like a bit more, there are lots of options! Use plenty of lube when you slide this in: she may even want to do it herself, if this is new for her, so she can set the pace. Once it's in, the plug should stay in place while your attentions are elsewhere. Use your mouth to stimulate her clitoris while you stroke her inside her vagina: with the butt plug this will feel extra-intense!

EDIBLE BODY PAINT

You've seen them in strange gift stores for years, why not try it out! Edible body paint is messy, but it can be a great way to start a wild and fun oral sexcapade. Have her draw out instructions (I'm thinking arrows, with maybe a bulls-eye or two), then you follow them. You can have a lot of fun with body paint! Draw on one another, then take turns kissing and licking it all off. If you're worried about the mess, minimize it by tossing down an old blanket, or playing in the bathroom, then hopping into the shower when you're finished!

KISSABLE BODY POWDER

Or try this classy and clean alternative to the edible body paint. Dust on this tasty powder, then devour her like a doughnut! Where body paint is sticky and messy, this powder is soft and pretty. This accessory is sexy and sensual, a perfect addition to a classy rendezvous. Even if your tryst isn't ringed with candles and accompanied by soft jazz, this stuff will class you up.

GOOD VIBES

෴

Why do we use vibrators as sex toys? As anyone who's ever sat on a misaligned washing machine can tell you, vibrations feel good. Your typical vibrator is a simple machine: most consist of a simple motor with an added weight that destabilizes it. As the motor runs, the added weight throws off the engine's balance, creating a "shimmy" or oscillation that your body feels as waves of vibration. These vibrations bring blood flow to the area, encouraging your tense muscles to relax and heal; this is why they're used in high-tech massage chairs. But when applied to an erogenous zone, especially one with such varying sensitivities as the vulva, vibrations pack an extra punch! The vibrations stimulate sensitive areas, bringing blood to the surface (making her more sensitive) and sending jolts of pleasure through her nerve endings.

Vibrators have a weird history for a sex toy: the first people to wield the devices were Victorian era doctors seeking to relieve their female patients from the pains of "hysteria," sometimes also called "wandering uterus," by stimulating their genitals until their ill health was relieved through a fit of "paroxysm." Hysteria was the term for a common female ailment of the time, one that we might call "mind-melting boredom that drove a bunch of upper-class ladies batshit insane." I give credit to everyone involved for deciding that the best cure for this boredom was orgasms, however they want to call them. Before the happy discovery of the vibrator, doctors had to relieve their patients by hand, a task that took some skill, and a tedious amount of time. Well-born women received treatment in their own homes, and it is thought that the lovely fainting couches or chaise lounges that were so popular through the Victorian era were used not for the swooning, corseted maiden, but were made to keep the lady comfortably reclined as her doctor got her off!

The vibrator has enjoyed varying popularity since its creation: it was quite a popular appliance until its association with porn made it more of a sex toy than a medical device. Technological advances and the sexual revolution lead to a revival in the 1960s, when for the first time, a woman could buy a cordless, home-use vibrator of her very own! From then on, vibrators have slowly become more acceptable, mainstream, and popular for women of all ages, appearing in popular TV shows and other media. Today you can probably find a vibrator at your local drugstore, right alongside the condoms and lube. Big condom companies run promotions where they hand out sex toys from a truck like some kind of grown-up ice cream man.

Vibrators aren't seen as just a smutty sex toy anymore. That's still a big part of it, of course! But even sex therapists often advise women who have trouble orgasming to pick up a vibrator to help with their self-explorations.

OUT OF THIS WORLD *HER* POSITIONS

THE ROYAL DINNER

This position is fit for a queen, all she has to do is lie back and let you do the work. Think of it as the missionary position of cunnilingus, the go-to starter move, and for good reason! At this angle as your mouth is focused on her clitoris, you have very easy access to her vagina, and she's in the perfect position for you to stroke her g-spot.

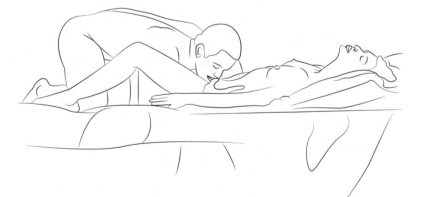

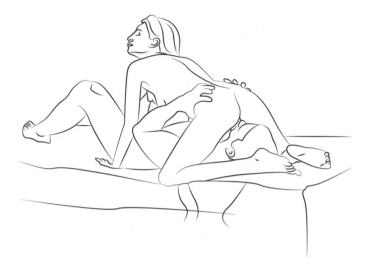

SHE'S ON TOP

Propped up on top, straddling your face, she has lots of control over the action. Lie on the bed and have her climb on top of you. Have her straddle your face, spreading her legs until she's lowered into place. She can stay on all fours or lean down on your torso, however is most comfortable. You get a new perspective, and a great view of her ass as you practice all your tricks. Follow her rhythm as she grinds against your mouth.

From this position your hands are free to roam. Use them to grip her hips and pull her closer, or squeeze her ass. She can also move freely: she can move closer or farther from your mouth, or pull away if it gets too intense, coming back when she's ready.

THREE-RING CUNNILINGUS

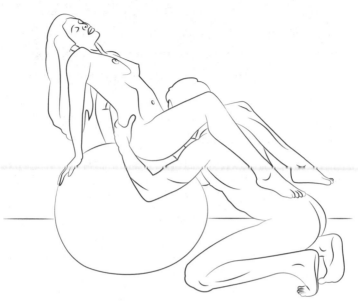

An exercise ball can add a fun balancing element to your oral play: if you have one handy, try this move. Or maybe it will inspire you to take up whatever exercises you're *supposed* to do on an exercise ball. Have her sit on the ball as you kneel in front of her. Rest her legs on your shoulders as you bring your face closer to her pussy. She can lean back and place her hands on the ball to brace herself, while you hold her hips to steady her and hold her close. She can bounce, thrust, and sway, using the gentle motion of the ball to give her another layer of sensation as you work your own magic.

If you don't have an exercise ball, try cunnilingus with her seated on a chair or on the edge of the bed, with you kneeling between her legs. The angle of this position puts more focus on the clitoris, and gives your partner plenty of opportunity to participate: she can move her hips to redirect your tongue, shift herself to set the rhythm, and if the spirit moves her, she can grab your head to directly increase the pressure! She's also got a great view of the show!

STANDING OVATION

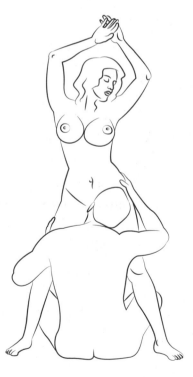

Good oral sex doesn't have to be horizontal: try this hot wall position when she wants to stretch her legs! Have her stand against a wall with her legs spread as wide as is comfortable. Arrange yourself between her legs: depending on your height, sit or kneel so your face is directly at pussy level. Move in close and wrap your hands around her hips and thighs to help steady her. Stroke, squeeze, and fondle her ass and legs as you go down on her. She can play with her tits, grip your head, or stand back and enjoy. This position is perfect for shower sex, as long as she can stay steady on her feet!

HULA GIRL

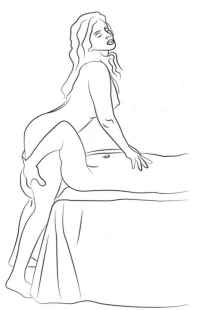

Can your girl spin a hula hoop? This position will have her moving her hips in no time! Recline on the edge of the bed, with your head hanging off. Have her stand at the foot of the bed, facing toward you, straddling your face. Have her move until she's in position while you help steady her with your hands. With her spread out above you, you have perfect access. She can shift her body to help you hit the right spot, and she has a great view of your work. Standing above you can help her feel in control: add some bondage, and you have a great scene for a starter dominatrix. Or maybe she just likes to hula!

NO-HAND HANDSTAND

If you want a challenge with an explosive reward, try this acrobatic position. Pick her up and hold her against you, facing away. She can wrap her arms back and around you for extra stability, but you really shouldn't be trying this if you think you'll drop her on her head! If you can manage it, the flipped orientation makes this position super stimulating.

If you're not quite ready to join Cirque du Sex, don't despair: this position can be easily modified into a kind of intermediate free-weights move. Have her lie back across an ottoman or a big pillow—anything big enough to prop under her and make her

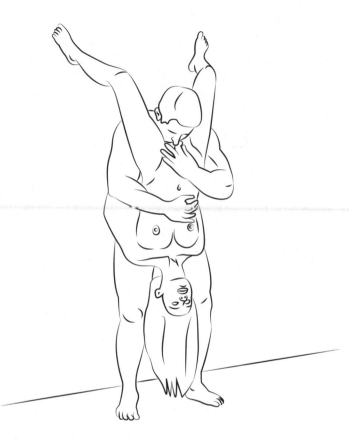

arch her back. Have her hang her ass off the edge of it. Set yourself up between her legs, then slide your arms under her thighs and grab her ass. Lift her up to meet your mouth and give her your best moves, then lower her down, squeezing and massaging her ass. Then do as many reps as you can!

Part Two

As the apple tree among the trees of the forest, so is my beloved among the men. With great delight I sat in his shadow, and his fruit was sweet to my taste.

—Song of Solomon 2:3

INTRODUCTION TO PLEASURING HIM ORALLY

All men love head, therefore all men love all head. False! Wrong! For the love of God, just stop. It is a rare man who will turn down fellatio, but there is more to giving great head than just gracing his penis with your presence. Whether going down is foreplay, coreplay, or both for you and your partner, it's important to know where you're going, where you want to take him, and how you plan to get there. With a quick brush-up on his anatomy, an ode to grooming, some kink, and of course the how-to, this section will go well beyond the need-to-knows of oral sex for him. Your downtown dexterity (and enthusiasm!) will be the difference between your guy just loving head—and your guy loving *your* head.

WHAT'S UP DOWN THERE: A GUIDE TO MAN PARTS ANATOMY

All too often, the penis is given all of the attention, while other zones that are just yearning to be touched, licked, teased, and sucked are neglected. Here is a list of some of the obvious and not so obvious zones of his manhood so that you can touch him in ways he'll fantasize about well after you've finished.

THE PENIS

This is your first problem: focussing on "the penis." His shaft is by no means one-dimensional (that would be a shame), both in terms of what he feels and how he feels it. So why do we talk about it as if it's a singular entity? All parts of the penis are not created equal, and as such, each part should be treated with special attention!

GLANS

The *glans*, coming from the Latin root word for "acorn," is the rounded tip of the penis through which men both urinate and ejaculate. In uncircumcised men, the glans is covered by the foreskin unless he is aroused. Whether your guy is circumcised or not, this is the most sensitive area of the penis, and therefore a part you should learn to know and love. Referring to it as the "glans" may sound a tad medical while you're talking about getting someone off, so society has presented us with all sorts of nicknames throughout the years: "mushroom tip," "head," "helmet," and "dome," just to name a few.

Like the beacon of a lighthouse signaling sailors in the night, the tip of his penis is a beacon for bliss that you're meant to pay attention to. Use your tongue to flick rhythmically against the head or massage sensuously. Vary your pace, and while you work your magic elsewhere, feel free to massage it with your lubricated hand to keep his tantric tempo way up. While this hot spot is the equivalent of the clitoris in its sensitivity to all that attention you're giving it, keep in mind that giving it *too* much attention can occasionally go awry. Just like any sensitive zone, unpleasant textures, dryness, and too much friction can be painful. While some people joke that "just the tip" doesn't qualify for having had sex, the same can be said for giving phenomenal head. Be good to the tip, but don't forget that this is just one of the stops (and not necessarily the first) on the road to oral ecstasy.

CORONA

Aptly named after the Spanish word for "crown," the *corona* is the rounded ridge where the head of his penis meets the shaft. As the circumference of the *glans*, the corona is packed with sensitive nerves that are ready to be teased and tempted by your tongue.

Use the tip of your tongue to run along this sensitive ring or flick rapidly to keep him on high alert.

This is a good area to tease lightly before you take him in your mouth, as well as an excellent go-to if you've been concentrating on one area for too long. While it's important to have a steady rhythm as you go down on him, switching things up will keep things from getting monotonous.

MEATUS

The *meatus* is the hole in the center of the tip of his penis. It's a little-known pleasure zone, that with some added pressure with your tongue, will add a little something extra to your repertoire. Keep in mind, though, that while it's a uniquely good feeling, it's no El Dorado of hot spots—spending lengths of time here poking your tongue at it will just be confusing for everyone.

FRENULUM

The *frenulum* is the small bulb of flesh right below his corona, connecting to the shaft of the penis. This tiny cluster of nerves is so rich with pleasure potential that it's a shame it's often overlooked. When you're tonguing down his shaft and head, take a moment to run your tongue along the circumference of his tip, and then flick rapidly on the frenulum. If you think you've done too much "flicking" as it is, put your lips at the bottom of his shaft, lightly gather the soft layer of skin with your lips and teeth (no biting!) using a little bit of suction, and glide your way up to his frenulum, continuing to suck lightly as you go. End this with a sensual kiss to the head of his penis before you make your next move.

FORESKIN

If the man in your life is uncircumcised, then you are familiar with his *foreskin*. This is the soft sheath of skin that covers and protects the *glans* when the penis is not erect. It is also a mucous membrane, much like the inside of an eyelid. When the penis is erect, the foreskin glides back over the penis to reveal the head.

Circumcision is popular in western culture, both for religious and health reasons. In the Book of Genesis (17: 10-14), Abraham instructs men to be circumcised and to have their newborn boys circumcised. As a result, circumcision has become one of the first celebrations for a newborn in Jewish families. On the eighth day after a baby boy is born, families celebrate the *brit milah* (pronounced "bris milôh" or just "bris"). The newborn is circumcised by a medically trained *mohel* (male) or a *mohelet* (female). While circumcision is not synonymous with Christian practices, New Year's Day is the holy day *Feast of the Circumcision of Christ* (according to the

Semitic calculation of days). In accordance with the Christian faith, this day accounts for the first drop of blood that Jesus shed for humanity.

In secular western culture, circumcision is generally performed to deter some of the health risks that can (but not always) come along with foreskin. The moist ecosystem under the foreskin can facilitate the spread of sexually transmitted diseases. However, and this is a big *however*, using protection and being a generally sanitary person about man care substantially decreases any of these risks, just as it would for a circumcised man.

While some talking (helmeted) heads like to argue that circumcision *is just so terrible! How dare you suggest I remove things from my amazing penis and subject me to a world devoid of pleasure!!!*, this is mostly just hubbub. There is no medical evidence to suggest that circumcision, when done properly, is harmful or negatively affects the penis's sensitivity. While much of this information seems like a cheerleading session for circumcision, many lovers of the uncircumcised man prefer the foreskin for its texture—the ribbed sensation along his penis can make it feel like he's doing two things at once while you're getting down and dirty.

Whether circumcised or un-, performing fellatio is generally the same in terms of your tantalizing technique. As long as you are paying attention to your partner's *oohs* and *ahhs*, the sheath doesn't affect his sword. Either way, there should be no stigma regarding the haves and have nots, because penises are wonderful.

SCROTUM

Ohhhh, the *scrotum*! This should be one of your very favorite parts of the entire head-giving process, especially because it's one of his. The scrotum is the soft sack of skin that is the mahogany treasure chest to his family jewels. This area is extremely sensitive, both on the surface of his skin and on the sperm-producing testes themselves.

Get ready to lick, suck, massage and tease this area. If taking his balls into your mouth isn't your thing, you should really reconsider. If you've reconsidered, asked the heavens, spoken with oracles, and summoned an old shaman to find peace with the term "teabagging," and it's *still* not your thing, then just make sure to substitute the pleasure he would feel from your warm and wet mouth over him with your lubricated warm hands instead. The slippery sensation over his balls and sack while you give him head will have him writhing in ecstasy.

SCROTAL RAPHE

The *scrotal raphe* is the formation in the center of the skin of his balls that looks like a seam. The "raphe" is a term used for several different parts of the body, like the *lingual raphe*, which is the seam of skin on the underside of the tongue.

His nether raphe—not unlike the rest of his balls—is supersensitive and craves its own oral attention. While you're down there, think of the raphe as a line from point A to point Bliss: using the raphe as a guide, run your moistened tongue from the very bottom of his balls along this pleasure line, all the way up to the bottom of his penis. The sensation of your tongue running along this line will have him trembling as he gets ready for more attention from you and your mouth.

PERINEUM

Just behind the scrotum and right before you get to his back end, the *perineum* is the soft space in between. Sometimes referred to as the "gooch" or the "taint" (because it t'aint your ass and it t'aint your genitalia), the perineum's hypersensitivity is unsurprising, as it connects two major erogenous zones: his package and his back door. This spot is often neglected, but it is brimming with euphoric potential.

One mistake oral novices make is not getting handsy or exploratory enough. Yes, you are performing a blow job, which inherently implies mouth-to-penis action. But skipping over the less conspicuous bliss spots would be a mistake—like only hitting the major tourist hubs while you're on vacation and missing the hidden local gems. Gently massage his perineum while performing oral, or get even saucier and use your mouth. Take his penis in your mouth to lubricate his shaft, and then continue to massage it with your hand or massage his balls while you tongue his perineum. This technique borders on the seriously naughty because it's just shy of his back end, which is suggestive of a whole other world of deep desires.

ANUS

Yup, the butthole; how sexy for you! While many are adverse to the idea, incorporating his back door is one of those earth-shattering things that will change his perspective on head forever. With regards to female anatomy, there is no secret g-spot back there that is guaranteed to make a woman come, other than indirect clitoral stimulation. Luckily for men, such a pleasure hub exists! The prostate glands are located on the opposite side of the anal wall. Because of this, men can achieve orgasm from anal stimulation without even a stroke or a lick to the penis.

While you're performing fellatio, consider using your hands to sensually massage his balls, slowly move to his perineum, and then gently insert a lu-

bricated finger into his anus. Multitasking is important, because for the man who wants his partner to
explore anal play but may not want to address it,
having your mouth on his cock at the same time is
a good enough excuse for why he's moaning, *Holy
shit, [your name here], that's so fucking good!* This
form of anal playtime is generally a last-stop-on-
the-road technique before you expect him to come
(which he'll do, explosively), and one that should be
performed by your non-dominant hand to avoid any
cross-contamination.

GROOMING GUIDE FOR HIM:
MANSCAPING

While many men choose to go au naturale with regards to grooming their manzones, it's becoming
more popular—if not expected—to do a little manscaping. Some downtown grooming, whether a basic
trim or a full waxing, can be a confidence builder for
you and a turn on for your partner. It also says something about you and how you perceive your own
sexuality; consideration of this area suggests that
you want to appeal to your partner, which in turn,
is incredibly sexy for the one who gets to view your
work. The idea that a little *thought* has gone into

your pubic appearance makes it all the more gratifying for your partner that you want to be engaging in those sexy exploits with one another.

No one should feel fettered by the grooming mandates of those around them (whether by a partner or a magazine), but it is important to consider your partner when deciding what works best for you, especially if he or she does the same in return. If your partner is a traditionalist who has a thing for Magnum P.I., a look of disapproval after you've gotten a Boyzillian shouldn't surprise you. At the same time, you shouldn't be violating your own personal preferences for manscaping; if your likes are a deal-breaker for your partner, you probably have more than just a manzone grooming conversation ahead of you. Ultimately, finding a method and an amount that makes both parties happy will make your sex life more sexessful. Experimenting with hair removal can even be a form of foreplay—trying out new looks as a couple can open you both up to be sexually exploratory in ways you hadn't been before.

How you manscape is entirely your prerogative as both a package and a pubic hair owner. With that in mind, though, there is a pretty important pillar to successful manscaping **if you plan on getting head** that applies across the board, whether you prefer a natural and rugged, *I-chop-wood-while-wearing-flannel* look; a freshly waxed, *I-could-be-a-porn-star-*

but-maybe-just-a-hot-model look; or somewhere in between:

BE THE COURTEOUS GENT

If you want your partner to be spending large amounts of time pleasuring your manhood, the least you can do is make the job a little easier. Unless your partner has a fetish involving the Amazon, no one wants to feel like they need a machete to chop their way through all that hair (and more than likely, you don't want anyone wielding one there either). If you think someone spitting out hair looks incredibly un-sexy, it's likely that your partner *feels* incredibly un-sexy while doing it. Be a courteous gent and avoid all that by tidying the excess beforehand. Even if you are partial to a masculine, natural look, using a trim-mer or scissors to cut away the peripheral pubic hair will maintain the aesthetic without making you look like you gave zero thought to your own sexuality. Apply this gentlemanly mantra to your grooming habits regularly.

THE FINER DETAILS

Below are the three main ways to get all Edward Scissorhandsy with your manzone. Try one, two, or all three!

The Trimmer Guy:

Keepin' it neat! Trimming is the most widely used method of manscaping by men. It maintains the natural look that we were all born with, which—hooray!—has not yet been stigmatized by pop culture in the way that pubic hair has been for women. If your preference is to trim, you have the option of using your everyday scissors or an electric beard trimmer. Scissors are simple, easy to use, and certainly get the job done, but if you are a perfectionist, they can leave an uneven trim. Electric trimmers have adjustable heads that will alter the desired length of your hair for a more even, sculpted look. There are brands of trimmers that gear specifically toward your manzone, but mechanically speaking, it is exactly the same as the one you may use on your beard. Just make sure to label them properly!

The Shaver Guy:

This is an art that women, with their long legs and svelte vaginas, have mastered. What women often forget to tell men, though, is all the pains they go through for personal maintenance. Shaving has a trifecta of positives: It's fast, inexpensive, and exfoliates so that your desired areas are left silky and smooth. The downsides are that regular maintenance can cause itching, unsightly red bumps, and the hair can grow back coarsely and quickly. Some men choose to shave the whole thing, which may feel more hygienic and can make your junk look bigger. Others choose to keep the natural patch and just shave their balls (For the man who likes his balls sucked, this will earn you points: *Oh, you're so considerate!*) If you're a shaver—whether you shave the whole thing, just your balls, or artfully sculpt a symbol off of a Lucky Charms box—here are a few steps that will help you along:

1. Don't dry shave.
2. Halfway through a hot shower, apply shaving cream or a thick conditioner to your desired area. With a sharp blade, shave downwards with the grain. Shaving upwards and against the grain will give you a closer shave, but may irritate your skin and make more ingrown hairs.
3. When toweling off, pat the area with a dry towel; do not rub, as it may irritate your skin.
4. Apply an unscented moisturizer on the area you shaved; this will lock in moisture and can help prevent ingrown hairs. Scented moisturizers contain alcohol, which can burn and cause itching.

The Waxer Guy:

Oh hello, Mr. Porn Industry Guy! Waxing among men has become more popularized by the adult film industry, but it is also popular among athletes, tattoo enthusiasts, and your Average Joe. Much like a woman's motivation for waxing, men wax because it leaves clean, smooth skin around your package while requiring fewer treatments. Keeping a clean shave can require daily maintenance, but waxing can keep you bare for weeks. Among athletes or gym-goers, stripping away the hair shows off muscle definition; men with tattoos can feature their art; and for the nonspecific waxer, this form of manscaping feels more hygienic than shaving and will make your manhood look bigger. While stores do provide at-home wax kits, it's advisable to see an esthetician regularly who will wax efficiently, provide the right aftercare and moisturizers, and also not get squeamish halfway through and leave you with a semiwaxed pubic zone.

ORAL SEXNIQUES TO TURN HIM ON

Oral sex (and sex in general) should be an arena of passion where you always, *always* employ the Golden Rule. Treat your partner with the same enthusiastic, pioneering, fervent rapture with which you want him to treat you. Giving head should be nothing if not erotic and fun, so be inquisitive about the things you try, communicate with each other about what feels good and what doesn't, and let pleasuring your partner be something that is inherently pleasurable for you. Always remember that being passionate with your guy and making him feel an ecstasy bordering on the volcanic is really fucking sexy, but it's also the threshold for reciprocation! These sexy techniques below highlight some of the hottest, most effective ways to give phenomenal head and get you inducted to his Blow Job Hall of Fame.

What to do with your . . .
. . . Mouth

THE MOUTHGUARD

Give your guy's dick some special attention from your luscious lips. As you're sucking him off, spread your lips over your teeth as if you were trying to pad them or make a very un-sexy "O face." You are essentially using your teeth to create a centralized, cylindrical pressure zone, without the nasty raking consequences. This gives you the opportunity to direct where you want him to feel this moan-worthy special pressure, the speed with which you do it, and for how long you care to employ it. Use your self-made mouthguard to go up and down his shaft with an even pace. Be careful to always keep your lips covering your teeth, lest you accidentally take this hot technique to extremely unpleasant places.

WALK THE LINE
(WITH YOUR TONGUE)

One of the nice things about human anatomy is that it sometimes has instructions all laid out for us, if only we were to take a moment to investigate. One such instruction manual is his *raphe*. Men are equipt with *perineal, scrotal,* and *penile raphes,* which are the seam-like lines of skin in the center of each of these areas. Starting at his perineum, take your pointed tongue and follow this pleasure line. Slowly lick from his perineum, up along the midline of his scrotum, continue up the center line of his shaft, and end with a sensual kiss to the head of his penis. This will taunt and excite his entire pleasure package all at once, which is a nice change of pace when head can sometimes revert to a one-thing-at-a-time game.

THE ZIPPER

Cautionary blow job lore tells us that teeth are the bringers of mayhem and torture. This is only the case if you are incredibly careless, have an involuntary bit-ing reflex when he pulls your hair while you're blowing him (seriously guys, stop this if you want to keep your dicks), or were highly misinformed and think the raking technique is where it's at. For a **SENSUAL** blow job addition that incorporates teeth, this technique is more of a naughty nibble. Start at the base of his shaft and lightly gather some of the fleshy skin on his cock with your lips, tongue and teeth. The efficacy of this does **not** involve biting; it's more a light suction with your teeth slightly parted as if they were a set of tracks for your mouth to move along. With wet lips, use this track to zip slowly up his shaft to his tip, using his sensitive skin as a guide. It's a uniquely pleasurable feeling he will find nowhere else!

MATH MAGIC

Let's work with exponents! Get his ecstasy up to the tenth power with some oral mathematics. Incorporate counting your "head bobs"—or every time you make a complete journey up and down his shaft—to your repertoire. Start by counting down from five: take him in your mouth, holding the base of his shaft with your hand, and suck him up and down five times with a steady, swift rhythm. Pause to massage his shaft with your hand, and then repeat with four bobs, then three, then two, and then one slow, long kiss. From here, perform the reverse: start with another slow trip down his shaft, all the way up to the original rapid five. When you've finished with this, use your hands to beat him off with a super quick rhythm. The cadence of this blow job method will have him at all systems go.

What to do with your . . .
. . . Hands

Performing phenomenal oral sex does not always mean that your mouth is the star of the performance. Amazing head has everything to do with what your hands are doing while you use your mouth to bring your guy past blissful borders. Use these simple techniques during each lusty lip lock with your man's package, and have him thinking, even when you're not around, about what you can do.

THE PSEUDO DEEP THROAT

Is it men, porn, or popular sex magazines that have perpetuated the deep throating craze? The reality is that even if you *can* deep throat your guy's entire penis in your mouth to give head like a porn star, you may not *feel* like it. When you are going down on your guy, one of the easiest ways to have his dick throbbing for more is to use your hand as an extension of your mouth. First, make sure you have his shaft slick with your saliva or a water-based lube. When you put your lips to his tip, form an "O" with your hands around his shaft. Keep your mouth and your hand going in tandem while you go up and down his hard cock. Using your free hand, cradle and lightly massage his balls for some sensory overload.

POPPIN' BOTTLES

Sometimes when you're sucking him off, you need a little breather. Take this opportunity to perform one of the most erotic ways to jack him off. With his dick super slippery from your saliva or a lubricant, use your dominant hand to slowly massage his dick. With medium pressure, move your hand up and down his shaft in a corkscrew motion. Incorporating this tantric twist is exponentially better than a simple up and down motion, as it varies the pressure he feels on different parts of his cock and has him feeling multiple sensations while continuing the slow rise to climax. As you twist up and down, feel free to change your focus area: Use the twisting motion on just the tip of his penis for a few seconds, followed by an increase in pressure as you quickly go back down the length of his shaft. Incorporate your mouth by continuing the corkscrew motion and sucking his dick at the same time.

KUNG FU GRIP

Sometimes a little pressure and pain can be deeply erotic. While you're giving him head, wrap your hand around the base of his shaft and slowly increase the pressure. Lick and suck the top half of his dick while you tighten as hard as you can. This sexy squeeze will intensify the sensations in the rest of his penis. Slowly move your tight fist up the length of his shaft and back down again. One of the reasons this is so hot, though, is that you are cutting off circulation and causing blood to engorge in one area. Be careful only to do this for a short period of time, and also gauge his reaction to the increase in pressure.

FULL BODY CARESS

This oral position is all mouth on his dick and all hands on his body. Take his stiff penis in your mouth and perform a slow, hands-free oral. With your free hands, run your fingers along all of his erogenous zones and caress your palms along his body. Start with hands along his knees and up to his inner thighs. As you're sucking him off, use a little pressure and smooth out a full hand in his pubic zone, even digging your nails in a little. Moving upwards, use one hand to palm his stomach, chest and nipples, and use the other to caress the insides of one of his wrists, forearm, and elbow. The feel of your touch on all of his sensitive spots while you are giving him head will be a full body, full euphoria scenario.

THE DOUBLE PLAY

Multitasking is one of the leading causes of orgasm! While giving him unbelievable head, be sure to jack him off and play with his balls at the same time. Working both erotic components simultaneously will have him completely at your mercy. Massage one ball at a time, or both in tandem as you have your mouth and other hand working up and down his shaft. Vary your pressure on his balls, press into his perineum, or even tug lightly on his scrotum.

THE BOUQUET

Here's one floral arrangement he'll never forget to give you. With one hand coming from either side, try scooping up his balls and grasping the base of his cock as if you were holding a big bouquet of flowers. Use your mouth to continue to give him an amazing blow job, and use your hands to gently massage the arrangement in your hands. The pressure of his cock and his balls in close quarters with your hands while you give him head will be an altogether new feeling.

Let your fingers graze against his *mons pubis*—the soft pad of skin over his pubic bone where his hair is (or isn't). Use your thumbs, which should meet at the underside of his shaft, to massage in circular motions. Incorporate your tongue with this tempo and continue to bring him to downtown bliss.

THE TWIN TWISTERS

This way to get a little handsy with your guy takes the corkscrew motion and calls for backup. When it's time to give your mouth a little rest, sit up straight while you kneel in front of him. Begin massaging his lubricated dick with both hands. Perform the twisting motion simultaneously with both hands, covering his entire shaft and the head of his cock. The twisting sensation on his tip will drive him wild, while your hands on his base and the rest of his shaft will keep him on an upward trajectory to an amazing climax. When he looks to see what you're doing (which he probably will), lock eyes and maintain eye contact while you jack him off. Watching each other while you pleasure one another will bring you both to a blissful boiling point.

What to do with his . . .
. . . Balls

WET AND WILD

Sex is messy, but blow jobs are messier. With this head technique (which you should really use as a touchstone for all head sessions), use your saliva to give him such phenomenal head that he won't be able to tell his cock from his balls. Give his shaft a tonguey rubdown so that he is completely slick. Take his balls into your mouth (one at a time is fine), getting them super wet. Use your hands and tongue to disperse the lubrication. Switch between sucking him off and sucking his balls: If you're sucking his balls, make sure to be massaging his shaft; if your mouth is on his shaft, make sure to be massaging his balls. Try bringing his shaft and his balls together and licking them down simultaneously. This glossy head session will be unlike any other if you follow a standard his and hers blow job mantra: If you're not completely covered in one another's juices, you're doing it wrong.

TUG O' WAR

Testicles are sensitive. Because we know this, head-givers the world over sometimes stray from experimenting with ball play because they are afraid of causing damage or making an unpleasant mistake. While this worry is a realistic one, such a fear shouldn't hinder the attention you give to his sack. While you're giving him head, cup his balls gently with one hand. Keeping your hand cupped, use the tips of your fingers to gather the top of his fleshy scrotum, and slowly begin to pull. With a firm hand, pull his orbs toward you as you use your thumb to gently thumb each one. His scrotum is packed with sensitive nerve endings, so the pulling sensation will be a uniquely erotic addition to the way you play with his balls.

What to do with his . . .
. . . Back Door

At the mention of anal play, some men are quick to clench their cheeks and start a macho diatribe about why only women are for ass-fucking. These men are idiots. If he wants an orgasm that will have him shooting his load across the room, a little attention can be paid to this sensitive area. Unlike a woman's rump, a man's back end is an erotic hub because it is located adjacent to his prostate, which means he can get off with just anal stimulation. While you may not want to devote an entire sexy session to *just* anal stimulation, it is an unbelievably hot step on the way to taking him to a mind-blowing orgasm.

THE PROSTATE MASSAGE

This is a stimulating addition to head-giving that he won't soon forget. As you're giving him head, begin by massaging his balls, making your way to his perineum. Gently run a finger from front to back, and rub around the outside of his asshole. With a lubricated finger, slowly insert it into his anus and rub gently. When your finger is a little less than halfway inside, make a "come hither" motion. This will stimulate the area around his prostate, and begin his trajectory toward climax. Continue to give him head while you do this, using your other hand to play with his balls or massage his shaft in tandem with your mouth.

ANALINGUS

It's the ultimate taboo. A not-for-everyone route, analingus is seriously naughty. (A disclaimer: Please shower, scrub, and soap each other up beforehand. Nobody wants to contract some weird ass disease, even if it is the one you love's weird ass disease.) Showering together is incredibly sexy, so get all riled up together as you taunt and tease with soap suds.

Dark was the night as pitch,
or as the coal,
And at the window out

she put her hole,
And Absolon, to him it
happened no better nor worse,
But with his mouth he kissed
her naked arse
Savoring it before he was
aware of this.
Back he jumped,
and thought it was amiss,
For well he knew
a woman has no beard.
He felt a thing all rough and long
haired,
And said, "Fie! alas!
what have I done?"
—Geoffrey Chaucer, *The Miller's Tale*

Whether you continue this technique in the shower or move to another locale, start by licking and kissing your guy all over. Run your fingers along the inside or back of his thighs, trailing this touch with wet kisses. Lick his shaft and balls, performing fellatio until you feel like moving on. Start with a descent to his perineum, and then use your flattened tongue along the inside of his cheeks. Make circular motions around his hole, or have him turn over and lick along his crack. Insert your tongue into his hole and choose your pace by flicking, moving slowly in and out, or moving it in circles. Keep things extra hot by continuing to jack him off or massage his balls at the same time.

Kink for Him

There's no doubt that the tools you were born with make their own amazing oral sex toys. As humans, though—from playing with fire to building skyscrapers—ingenuity, the curiosity to improve the seemingly unimprovable, and the concept that anything with batteries is automatically more fun, has led us to build a fantastic industry: Sex merchandise. Below is a list of toys, tricks, and treats to take your playtime from fucking hot to fucking hot and kinky.

DEEP THROAT SPRAY

For those of us head-givers who were not blessed with an immunity to large objects being rammed into our throats, there is a numbing spray out there to help! Generally sold in peppermint and cinnamon flavors, deep throat sprays are a numbing agent that you spray at the back of your throat to help deter your gag reflex. Spray one to three squirts and wait a few seconds to let the numbing set in. Be prepared for a little discomfort at first, as a numb throat can sometimes trick your brain into thinking you are having trouble breathing. The numbing spray will help you take your man's dick farther into your mouth, but the degree to which this is effective will entirely depend on your comfort level, the size of your mouth, and the size of his penis. Don't spray directly onto his penis, as numbing his cock will completely defeat the purpose of giving him head in the first place!

HOT AND COLD

Sensation play is an easy (and free!) way to spice up your oral sex life. Using ice and a cup of hot water or tea, tempt and tease his cock by changing the temperature of your mouth. Start by biting an ice cube and trailing it along his lips, down his neck and torso, and all the way to his package. Make him shiver all over as the ice melts coldly against his hot skin. Ease the freeze by switching between the ice and your lips and mouth, and when the cube is gone, keep the oral game going. Take a couple of sips of hot tea and let it return the heat to your mouth from the chill of the ice. Swish or let it settle until your mouth and lips are warm and ready for him. Bring your steamy self to his cock and begin kissing, licking, and taking him into your mouth to bring his temp from the arctics to the tropics. Go back and forth between these two sensations to make a long-lasting sexy session.

ORAL MINTS

These peppermints are a great way to give a fantastic blow job with a plethora of kinky sensations. The intense minty flavor along his shaft will have his dick tingling with excitement. Play with the mints in two ways: First, try crushing the mint up in your mouth right before you go down on him. The crushed mint will disperse along your tongue and over his shaft so that he can feel this minty tingle all over. For a different feel, take a whole mint and place it on the center of your tongue. As you take him in your mouth, treat the mint like a pleasure beacon. Massage the underside of his shaft with your tongue, while the hard mint adds a stiff pressure button to your oral fun. Move the mint to the other side of his shaft (and therefore to your upper lip or roof of your mouth) to add the pressure to this less often attended area. The stiff nub will radiate a cool minty feel that will bring an exciting new element to your blow job repertoire.

FIZZING ORAL CANDY

This powdery oral candy will sizzle, fizz, and pop in your mouth as you go down on your guy and give him an extra tingle. Much like the candy you know and love from growing up, this cherry-flavored fairy dust is intended to send his BJ skyrocketing. How much fizzle he'll feel in his swizzle depends on his dick's sensitivity, but it's never disappointing to try out a sexy new treat! Pepper it onto his cock while you're getting naughty, licking it off to get him snapping, crackling, and popping his way to sexy heights. Alternatively, try dusting some in your mouth before you begin so that the fizzing is well under way by the time you start your oral choreography. Just maybe skip the swish of Coke while you're down there.

VIBRATING COCK RING

Women have been enjoying vibrators for a century now, but it was only a matter of time before men figured out just how good these vibrations could be. A typical cock ring is a silicon ring that is slipped on tightly to the base of a man's erect penis. The squeezing sensation entraps some of the blood flow so that your guy can maintain his erection significantly longer. The *vibrating* cock ring is exponentially more fantastic. The ring will have a large nub on one side that has two functions: It acts as both a clit tickler (awesome) and the on/off switch for the replaceable watch-sized battery. Lube up your man's penis with a water-based lubricant or begin to give him head to make him nice and slick. Click the on switch and slide the ring (nub-face up) down his shaft to the base of his penis. Lick, suck, and massage his penis while he experiences the vibrating ring tight around his cock. Your amazing blow job combined with the vibrations throughout his whole package will bring him to an extra-long, high-intensity climax. The best part of this kind of oral is that you can switch back and forth from a blow job to traditional intercourse. Blow jobs shouldn't always be one-sided, which is why the benefits of such a cock ring are great for couples; the blissful buzz will send you into a heated overdrive right alongside him. Many manufacturers promise up to 80 minutes of buzz for you and your guy, which can be dispersed among many sexy sessions or one hot marathon.

OUT OF THIS WORLD
HIM
POSITIONS

THE HANDSTAND

You sexy acrobats, you! This position requires extensive balance and upper body strength by him, and the ability to stand by you. While he may be exerting exorbitant amounts of energy while you casually stand in front, the payoff for him is that—*oh right!*—he is getting his dick sucked. He should perform a steady handstand against a trusted wall (partitions made of rice paper with paintings of calming bonsai trees are not recommended), perhaps putting a soft mat on the floor to lessen the tension on his hands. Keep in mind that as you perform fellatio, his penis will be at the opposite angle as a traditional blow job. As you stand, lower your back and bring his penis upwards or kneel down to take his penis in your mouth from below. With such an open stance, he is presenting himself as a smooth canvas for you to kiss, lick, and massage without instruction or interference. By exerting so much energy and letting the blood rush to his head during this erotic blow job, these all-consuming sensations will heighten the intensity he feels on his dick. Be wary of reaching a climax in this position, though, as it may weaken his arms and send him headfirst to the floor.

THE HOLY GRAIL

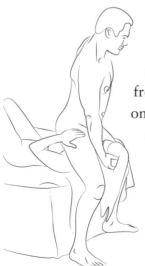

This position is a fellatio switcheroo, which requires very little effort from you, and slow, erotic thrusting from him. Lie perpendicularly on the bed, while he straddles above you. Gently cupping your head and the back of your neck to prevent tension or strain, he performs *irrumatio*, which is essentially reverse fellatio. The term "fellatio" refers to you performing oral pleasure on a man, who remains passive, whereas "irrumatio" means that you are passive and the man performs the motions of oral sex. He should be sure to keep a slow, sensual pace, so as not to hurt or gag you. You can use your tongue and mouth to sensually lick and suck his penis as he glides in and out. At the same time, you can run your fingertips up and down his thighs, balls, backside, arms and chest to heighten his excitement. This position transforms a run-of-the-mill blow job into a sexy interactive event.

THE CROSSROADS

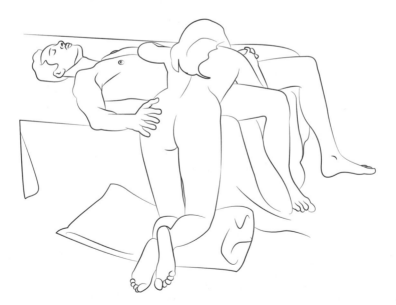

Meeting a crossroads doesn't have to be a life-changing event, but it can definitely change the way you think of giving phenomenal head. He lies down on the bed with his feet resting on the floor. You kneel on the floor perpendicularly to him (i.e. you should be facing the horizontal view of his abdomen). This angle allows your mouth to glide down his penis at a different angle from traditional fellatio, which will let your tongue explore those surfaces of his shaft that are needy for attention. This angle also gives you free rein to caress his legs and massage his balls, while presenting the opportunity for him to clutch your ass to ride along his pleasure trajectory.

TWO FOR ONE

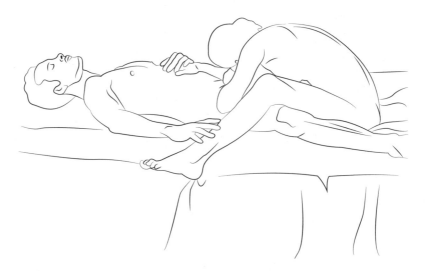

Oral sex doesn't have to be the main event; it should also be used as foreplay to make your lusty session all the more mind-blowing. In this position, he lies down on the bed as if you were performing traditional fellatio at his waist below. The difference here is that your legs straddle his hips so that you are at the ready to pounce on his dick when you so desire. This does require a little flexibility on your part, as you'll be slouched over his package as if you were trying to touch your nose to the floor at yoga. The great thing about this sexy straddle is that you get to take control and be a little selfish with your own pleasure needs. As you give him head and get him riled up, visualize what it'll feel like to be riding on top of him to get yourself hot and bothered. When you feel like joining the fun, spring up and slide yourself onto his shaft to ride each other into ecstasy. To add a kinky twist, switch back and forth between giving him head and fucking him; he'll think it's super hot that you're tasting your own flavor while you tongue him down.

BALL BLISS

Count giving your guy oral bliss as your exercise for the day! Using an exercise ball, have him sit centered on the ball as he awaits your oral gift. Kneel down between his legs, teasing him by running your fingers from the insides of his feet, around his ankles, and up the insides of his thighs. Follow this soft touch with your pouted lips and light, tonguey kisses. You'll be able to tell how well you're teasing him by how bouncy that ball starts to get. As you make your way to his package, lightly kiss the insides of his pelvis, bringing your tongue to his balls. While he controls the exercise ball, you'll control his: Lightly cradle his testicles with soft hands and take them into your mouth, being sure to move your tongue around them in a sensual massage. Quickly move from doing this to moistening his shaft with your mouth, and as you return to sucking his balls, massage his now wet penis with your free hand. The two sensations at once will feel incredible for him and exciting for you as you watch his reaction. Just be careful—the more he likes it, the more the ball will bounce and potentially gag you (and you can save ballgags for another time!).

Part Three

Us

Now that you're both certified in the art of oral sex, it's time to put it all together. Oral sex is a great addition to a couple's sex life: as foreplay, or as the main event, oral sex helps ensure that both partners are satisfied and enjoying themselves, something that's harder to guarantee during penetrative sex. Where penetrative sex lets you use your body to give and take pleasure, oral sex has you focused on your partner's most intimate parts. If you're both feeling frisky, you can still enjoy the biggest (non-)bang for your buck, you just need to be creative!

MASTURBATION CRASH COURSE

If you plan on pleasuring each other, you should first know how to pleasure yourself. This is a Do It Yourself (Together!) discussion of the pros and cons of getting yourself off. Masturbation doesn't have to be an act performed in solitude, either; watching how your partner likes to get off is a window into their secret pleasures, and it's also like your own little homemade porno!

Unlike the scare tactics from early adolescence, masturbation won't make your palms hairy, and it probably won't make you go blind, but there are some pitfalls of handling your own bacon too often. If you're just getting down in one way, you may be conditioning your body to respond to only a specific kind of stimulation. This problem can get wrapped up in your porn watching habits, but the issue is primarily mechanical. When young men and women learn to masturbate quickly and furtively, when no one is looking, and all the while dreading anyone catching them, we get men and women who know how to masturbate hard and finish fast. Men can get what we call an "iron fist": they masturbate so hard and so often that they have trouble feeling pleasure or reaching orgasm from their partner's caresses. Women are not immune to this: some women may have sensitivity issues if they are often stimulating their clitoris directly with a powerful vibrator. In this case, too, bad masturbation habits get people hooked on super stimulating, wham-bam-thank-you-ma'am orgasms that are mostly sizzle and no steak. And the solution is more masturbation!

But instead of quick, adolescent masturbation, you're going to enjoy grown up, partnered masturbation. The goal is to reprogram yourself to get more pleasure out of subtle touches and strokes. You can do this when you're playing solo, too: slow it down, and let your hands explore. Don't try to orgasm right away, just try to feel good. Get to know what your body likes, and you'll have more fun with and without a partner.

MASTURBATION INSPIRATION

Need some help getting your fingers moving? Don't worry about stage fright, you just need some motivation! People like to say "men get off this way" and "women get off this way," and while there might be trends one way or the other, how you get off has more to do with you and less with your gender. I think everyone can benefit from classier, better-quality porn, so here are some ideas that you might like better than a three second preview on that seedy Internet porn site.

ARTSY PORN

Did you know you can find naked pictures on the Internet!? Of course you did, because the Internet is overflowing with porn. But did you know that some of it is actually good? "Good" is clearly a statement of opinion, but you can find sites that take a more artistic approach to their work. Good lighting and camera work and natural and healthy-looking models make for a more sensual experience, so keep your pinky up and call it *erotica*, not porn. You can find curated collections on sites like Tumbler and Pinterest, or you can find sites that produce and distribute their own high-quality erotica. I recommend *X-Art*, at www.x-art.com, for some very pretty porn! They also have videos!

ROMCOM WITH A TWIST

If you'd prefer your porn to be a talky, try finding videos with a more story-focused bent. A romantic comedy can get your sex imagination running better than a clip of some guy "delivering pizza" or "fixing the refrigerator." There are plenty of higher-quality pornos out there if you're willing to look for them, but a good place to start is The Romance Series, a site that specializes in creating erotic videos focused on romantic storytelling and realistic sex scenes.

READY READER

Remember when that certain monochrome erotic novel hit it big, and everyone started calling it "Mommy Porn" and acting all astonished that women like smut? I have a secret for you: erotic romance has been enjoying a revival lately, and that book's success only made it bigger! With e-books and online purchasing, buying and reading smut has never been easier or more private. And there are stories tailored to every taste, whether you dig werewolves and vampires, futuristic lesbian sci-fi, tough-talking lawyers, strong yet emotionally vulnerable firefighters, or anything in between, there's a book for you. If you're not a big fan of visual porn, erotic romance could be your style. Even if you enjoy porn in general, you may find written erotica stimulating in a whole new way. Reading porn you have to engage your imagination, and paint your own fantasies. Reading erotica, by yourself or with your partner, can help you explore your fantasies and build up a ready supply of inspiration for when you're getting off! You can find erotica all over the Internet: there are plenty of sites that offer erotic fan fiction, and erotic romances of all genres. Check out Literotica.com for some popular user-submitted stuff. If you want something a bit more polished, check your local book store or e-book store for published erotica. My friends at Ravenous Romance have provided some excerpts from bestselling authors Jennifer Dellerman and Cat Johnson!

RAVENOUS ROMANCE EXCERPTS

HOT LICKS
BY JENNIFER DELLERMAN

In this excerpt, Gwen and her mate Rome enjoy some intimate time after escaping a group of dangerous pursuers.

Without waiting for permission, Rome lowered his lips to her astonished ones. Perfect. He plunged his tongue deep into the wet, velvet heat of her mouth, tasting her sweet essence. He knew from that first kiss he could get lost right here, drinking her in. His cock swelled under a heavy wave of arousal, his veins felt thick with molten lava, fueling his desire. Deepening the kiss, he swept his tongue against hers, coaxing the response he craved.

Then Gwen was kissing him back, her hands curling on his bare shoulders, her tongue delving into his own mouth. Lowering his hands, he cupped her breasts. Generous, they had easily filled his palms last night and he'd ached all night and day to have those soft globes fill them once again. More than that, he wanted them in his mouth.

Reaching back, he unhooked her bra, catching the warm weight of her breasts as they sprang free from their confinement.

A faint moan of need trembled in her throat, the sound filling him with elation. He kept kissing her, tasting her as he alternated between kneading her breasts and lightly pinching the nipples that thrust hard into his palm.

The rough gasp she made spurred him on.

His mouth moved lower, nibbling, leaving a trail of hot, open-mouthed kisses along her neck. He drew her bra away just in time for his lips to wrap around one turgid nipple. Her fingers were in his damp hair, her short nails digging into his scalp as she pressed him closer. Shifting to take her other breast into his mouth, he teased her first with a long lick, then he parted his lips to draw her in, sucking strongly, elevating her arousal with the flick of his tongue, the rough glide of his teeth.

When she was shaking, he widened his stance, lowering himself so he could explore the soft curve of her belly. He dipped his tongue into her naval. Drawing in a deep breath, he scented everything Gwen. Her feminine arousal was a siren's call, making the blood pound in his cock. A pang of hunger so sharp and brutal he could barely think straight.

"Rome?" His name was an uncertain whisper and he looked up, knowing full well he couldn't hide the heightened state of lust that glowed in his eyes.

"Let me." It was more command than question, though he did manage to halt his downward slide to heaven long enough to give her time to tell him no. Not liking that possibility, he tacked on in a rough growl, "don't tell me no, bella. Please." At that moment he would beg on bended knee, offer up all his wealth and eternal obedience for a taste of her honey.

Her face flushed, her heaving chest causing her breasts to bounce enticingly. When
she pushed on his chest he nearly roared out
in angry frustration, but it was only to move
him back a fraction so she could inch to the
edge of the step.

He nearly fell to his knees in relief.

Cupping her face, he kissed her, pour-
ing out all he had into each brush of their
tongues. One hand circled to the back of her
head, the other her waist, as he leaned over
her, urging her to lay back on his shirt. He
never took his lips from hers as he stretched
one hand out blindly, seeking her own shirt.
When his fingers closed over the material, he
bunched it under her head, protecting that
part of her body from the hard, wide stone
step. And while he worried about her back,
she made no protest, no whimper of pain,
and he silently promised her that next time he
would lay her out over a thick, soft mattress.

He actually trembled as he took another
slow journey down the length of her body,
amazed by the smooth texture of her skin and
the toned muscles that flexed under his hand,
his lips. Catching her thighs in his hands,
he spread them further apart and settled his

mouth against the soaked cotton of her panties. He glided his teeth gently over the swollen flesh of her pussy, glorying in the way she arched her hips, the startled cry of pleasure that filled the air. He could taste her through the damp material. Taste her and crave more.

With an impatient growl, he snapped the sides with one sharp claw, thankful that cat shifters weren't like wolf shifters and could manipulate partial changes. For a short period of time at least, and usually reserved only in the case of an emergency.

To Rome, getting his mouth on Gwen's cream constituted an emergency. Of epic proportions.

His mouth clamped over her, his tongue diving in deep into her wet core. Not the gentle lapping of a kitten or the tender coaxing of a tentative lover. No, Rome was all fierce, primitive male, licking at her with long rasping strokes, giving pleasure as he luxuriated in her response. He wanted to roll around in her scent, crawl inside and let her surround him. As her feminine essence slid down his throat he felt his gums begin to burn. A warning that his fangs were about to descend without his permission, a harsh reminder that Gwen was his mate, and the cat jumping and clawing at the cage of Rome's control wanted her as much as the man.

A COWBOY FOR CHRISTMAS BY CAT JOHNSON

He supported her with a hand on each cheek of her ass. "Not that I'm complaining, but what got into you?"

"You." She planted a hand on each side of his face and kissed him, deep and thorough.

With a groan he picked her up. She wrapped her legs around his waist as he walked them both to the bed.

He laid her on the mattress and rolled to lie on his side as he gazed down into her face. "If this is the welcome I'm going to get, maybe I'll let the stragglers loose and go round them up again tomorrow."

"Sounds good to me." She pushed him onto his back and unbuckled his belt. He smelled of leather and horse and the outdoors.

"Let me take my chaps and boots off." Bonner moved to sit up.

"Oh no. Those stay on. The spurs too."

His eyebrows shot up, but he laid back down without complaint. It took a bit of doing, but she freed his cock from the fly of his jeans, while leaving the rest of his clothes on. Casey leaned low. She took the length of him between her lips and tasted the salty flavor of him.

Bonner groaned, low and deep in his throat. "Damn, girl. Are you living out some city girl-cowboy fantasy with me?"

Casey lifted her head. His length slipped out of her mouth with a pop. "Yup. That a problem?"

"Nope." He reached out and nudged her head down gently. "Go right ahead."

She did, lowering her mouth over his cock while making sure her teeth grazed him the whole way down. He was hard and smooth, like steel covered in satin. Bonner hissed a sharp breath and tangled his hands in her hair.

She lifted off him again, using plenty of teeth, and glanced up. "I like rough."

"Me too." Bonner's hold on her head tightened and he thrust into her mouth. That was the last talking they did for a while.

OUT OF THIS WORLD
US
POSITIONS

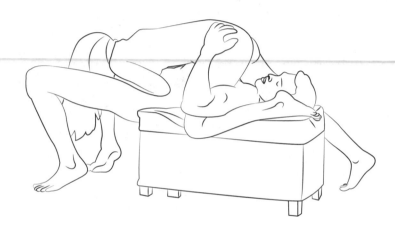

THE REVERSE HOOKUP

This steamy 69 is great for when you're just too hot for each other to find a bed. Using the ottoman in front of your couch or another padded surface, he lies down so that his whole back and head are rested and his legs are steadied in a 90 degree angle on the floor. She crawls on top of him, letting her tits graze over his mouth as she makes her way into position. This girl-on-top oral stance gives him a great view of her from below, and gives her easy access to his package from above. Since his legs and pelvis will be off the ottoman, his movement won't be hindered and he can rotate his hips in a slow, circular motion or thrust upwards gently as she licks him down. With her hovering right above him, he has an all-access pass to her pleasure zone and can lick, rub, suck, and finger her into ecstasy.

THE LAZY 69

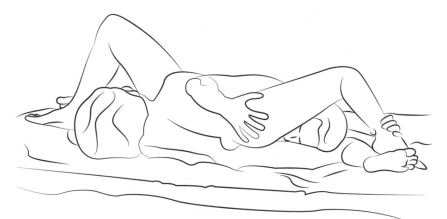

Whether you want it in the morning or on a rainy afternoon, this position is for when you're feeling super hot, but not super active. This sideways 69 lets you lie together in bed and worship each other's naughty bits with slow caresses, gentle kisses, and low, pleasured moans. On your bed or floor, pull each other in closely to a full-bodied embrace. He can massage her thighs and ass while she runs her fingertips along his side and the inside of his pelvis in a mutual tease. While your bodies are still and comfortable, put your energy into a deep makeout session with your partner's goods. Make your kisses and licks wet and slow so you bring one another to deep pleasure and throbbing bliss. When you both are so filled with erotic excitement that all you can feel is your rising climax and all you can hear is your heart pounding in your ears, tighten that full-bodied embrace, dig your fingers into each other's skin, and make this oral euphoric.

MASSAGE ENVY

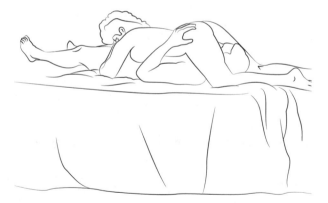

There is more to mutual head than just getting each other off in tandem. To take this already erotic act to sensual and slippery heights, make it a his-and-hers massage event as well. With hot oils or pleasant creams, rub each other down with your hands while you lick each other down with your tongues. As she lies on top of him, he can make her slippery in more places than one. As he licks her pussy, he should start by extending his arms above his head and rubbing the undersides of her feet. Bringing his arms lower, he can rub her oiled calves, her soft thighs, and her haunched rear end. When he's reached her pleasure hub, he should slip his fingers inside her while he uses his tongue. As he goes, she can use the same oils to rub his sides, slowly tease his knees and inner thighs, put pressure on his lower abdomen, and bring her warm and lubricated hands to his penis to jack him off and tongue him down at the same time. 69ing meets massage therapy as you two glide your slick bodies over one another and work out all of your oral tension!

DOWNWARD DOG

Sometimes being naughty means heading to uncharted territory. The best way to start with any bad girl or bad boy zone is by joining each other in the shower for a hot makeout session and some serious soaping action. When you've gotten squeaky clean and beyond horny for each other, take it to the bed.

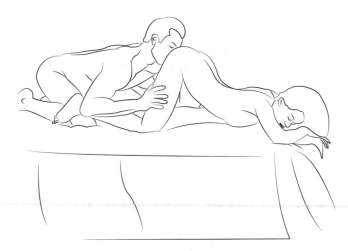

Back end bliss is gender neutral, so this position can apply to either partner. The receiver lies face down on the bed, with an arched back and pristinely presented rump. The arched angle and heightened ass is an optimum position for anyone ready for action. The giver should start slowly, especially if this is a first-time event. Begin by hovering over your partner, giving soft, tonguey kisses along the insides of his or her ankles, moving upwards along the calves, the inside of the knees, and up to the inside of the thighs. Move your hands along these areas too, but with an extra light touch to send shivers up your guy or girl. Bring those kisses to just below their ass, up their cushioned cheeks, and into their pleasure crevice. If you choose to start with traditional head first, that will get your partner really going, but don't do the reverse (moving from back end to front end can cause health risks for your partner). You can use a firm, pointed tongue or a soft, flat one while you work this area. Lick teasingly along their crack and in circles around the hole. If you want to be thorough, insert your tongue and massage your partner's front end goods at the same time. The dual naughty action will bring your guy or girl to a peak.

LICKING SKYWARD

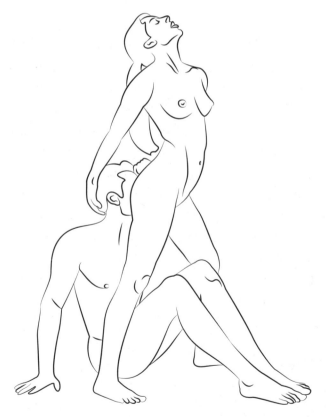

In a position where darkness and light come together, one partner looks to the naughty back door while the other looks to the pleasure heavens. This position can work two ways: If you and your partner aren't comfortable with anal play, it can act as foreplay without crossing that back door line. If you are totally into it, then follow this lead: The receiving partner stands with his or her legs parted, ready to be pleasured. As the giver, you should sit comfortably below and behind your partner's ass. Use this seating arrangement to do double duty: while you use your mouth, run your hands up your partner's legs and pleasure them from the front as well. Tongue his or her back side before you head right for anal play. Especially if you used a cleansing shower as foreplay, don't hold back! Introducing your partner to a new side of oral pleasure will bring an entirely new kind of lust into your already steamy relationship. This sitting giver doesn't have to be the only one in charge. The receiver will have full frontal access for personal pleasure or, if your partner is just too excited, can sit right down on top of you for some sexy intercourse.

THE UPSIDE-DOWN 69

This position is intense, for both partners. She's in the best position to give him deep-throat action, and he's got her all laid out in front of him. This is a passionate move, for when you can't get enough of each other! It may be difficult to give directions in this position (plus your mouths will be full), so make sure you're paying attention to your partner's body to make sure you're giving them what they want. If he's too heavy on top, have him prop up on his elbows and knees. Keeping her knees up, she can make sure he never leans on her too hard: she can arch her back and push him up with her body if she gets uncomfortable!

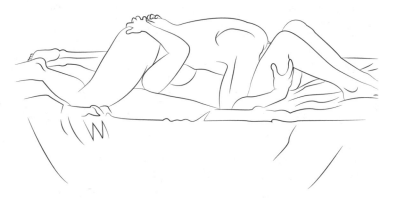

While you're rolled up together, take your time to use your hands as well as your mouth. Take a break from going down to kiss and stroke your partner. You have tons of erogenous zones within your reach, so let your hands explore, rubbing your partner's legs and back and squeezing their ass. Try to create as many sensations as you can, before you have to come up for air!

MISUSE OF FURNITURE

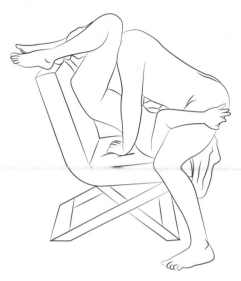

Are you eyeing that chair in the corner? The down-side of this position is you have to find the right furniture to pull it off, so you'll just have to try all of the chairs in your house until you find the one. I would recommend against that precariously balanced saucer chair. Or anything with wheels!

Once you've found your seat, help her into a semi-headstand, with her feet perched on the top of the chair and her head hanging off the seat. Move into position, with him leaning over her. She can wrap her arms around his legs to keep from slipping, and he can lean on the chair for support, depending on his height!

SOIXANTE-NEUF!

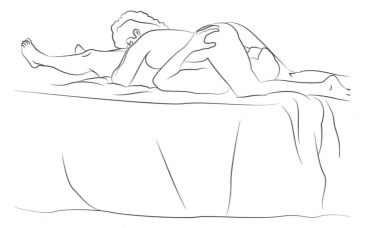

This is the most basic form of the 69 position, or soixante-neuf if you want to be all French about it. From this position both partners can rock their newly-honed skills (you did just read the rest of this book, right?) at the same time! Position yourselves comfortably, so you can reach your partner easily and touch where you'll want to. If you're the lady on top, try to resist the urge to be up on your knees: you may need to lift up a little to accommodate different-sized partners, but try to keep your body close to his. This lets him apply a bit more pressure, and makes it a bit of a different up close encounter. While he's at work, she can go down on him from above. This angle makes it easier for her to deep-throat, but she can also use her mouth on the head of his cock while her fingers slide over the shaft.

STRONG MAN

I think successful completion of this move should win you some kind of medal. There are a few ways to accomplish this, but however you do it, don't drop her on her head. You can start in the same position as on page 103 and scoop her up, or perhaps have her do a handstand and pick her up. Once you're in place, she can help hold herself up by locking her legs over his shoulders and wrapping her arms around his torso. He should keep his arms locked around her torso at her waist, and you should probably be standing on or near something soft to fall on. If you can get it up this position is thrilling! His adrenalin is pumping, which increases his pleasure, while she gets to feel him going down while she's upside down. Put this on your sexcapades bucket list, but maybe don't try it when you're drunk!

34 ½

I don't always like to 69: if I'm really jonesing for him to go down, I want his attentions on me, not distracted by my superb blow job skills. This move meets you halfway: whether she's already come or she just enjoys his manual skills, this position will keep both partners busy. She lays on the bed with her knees up and her legs spread. He straddles her face and she helps him get into position. This angle is great for deep penetration, but try to let her control the thrust depth and speed. Her hands can roam to fondle his balls and ass as he strokes her.

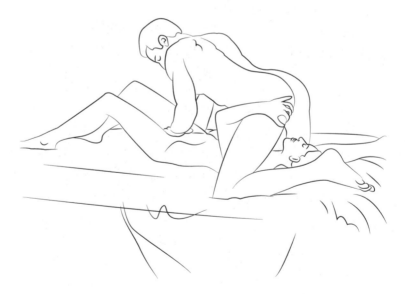

ORAL SURPRISES

Giving and receiving head can get old if you keep doing it the same way. Every once in awhile, make sure to try something new or be spontaneous—even if that "spontaneity" is completely planned!

SEXT MY DICK, BABY

Sexting is a super hot way to get each other riled and ready to pounce. When you have a few free minutes to get a little verbal, send a sexy text to your partner during his or her workday. Sexting during work can feel a little naughty because there is the fear of coworkers noticing rapid texting and those flushed cheeks (or a raging boner), but the payoff is amazing. Tell your partner how much you want to be giving them head, where you want to put your mouth, or give some sexty compliments. You'll both be squirming your way through your workday until you can get home and give them an unrivaled, passionate blow job.

LET ME PENCIL YOU IN

When your guy or girl has left the room, snag his or her smartphone or calendar and schedule a steamy oral session. Sign your name and write an insight to what you want to do, like "7:15PM–swirl my tongue over your tip," or keep it simple with "6:30AM–Mouth Fuck Each Other!" (Also, don't be an asshole with their phone; resist the urge to look through more than just your 7PM hummer.) Finding the oral date stamped in their calendar will make it one appointment they won't want to cancel.

GIFTS!

Buy your partner a gift card to a sex toy website or a sexy lingerie store. Peruse through the options together and set few limits to what they can buy. If you're going to set a limit, have it be something exciting, like that they can only choose a toy with batteries or something that can only be used on them. (If a gyrating dildo chair is something you've already said no to, this should be a previously accepted limit.) Many websites have sections entirely devoted to oral sex, so he or she can choose from an array of lubes, candies, edible underwear and toys. If you're at a clothing store, crotchless panties or silk ties can be a great way to get visual before you get oral.

LINGUAL LUNCH BREAK

Surprise your partner with a mouthy meal. Whether you show up unannounced at work (not always advisable), or schedule a lunch date together, take this date to the next level by ordering some hot oral for dessert. Do it in the car, the bathroom, or in a sequestered area where no one will stumble over you; whatever your locale, this will be an amazing midday surprise to get you both through the afternoon lull!

NUTRITION FOR HIS AND HER SEXUAL HEALTH

ᡣ

There is no magic superfood that will have your lady juices or man jizz tasting like the nectar of the gods, give you stamina that will have you riding each other all night, or make you the King or Queen of erotic pleasure. There are, however, several different foods that can at least make strides in those directions. To the chagrin of lazy people (i.e. everyone), only a well-rounded, healthy diet filled with lean meats, fruits, vegetables, and small amounts of red wine and chocolate are the key to staying healthy, both physically and sexually. The reality is, not exercising and filling your body with shitty foods will make you feel shitty, and that will ultimately manifest itself as weak stamina and low libido through poor blood flow to the genitals.

CARDIOVASCULAR HEALTH IS SEXUAL HEALTH

Unsurprisingly, if your heart is healthy and your circulation is flowing smoothly, so too does your sexuality. With proper circulation, blood flows to harden the penis and maintain a satisfying erection. Blood flow is equally important for women so that they can become engorged, lubricated, and ready for pleasure. Lower your intake of carbohydrates, unhealthy fatty foods, and make sure to work up a sweat for at least 20 minutes a few times a week.

WHAT'S IN YOUR NUTS AND FISH
Walnuts, Almonds, and Salmon, Oh My!

Arginine: Present in many healthy foods, arginine helps your body produce nitric acid. Nitric acid sets off neurotransmitters in your brain that tell the blood vessels in your genitals to expand, which helps his penis become erect and helps lubricate and engorge her vagina. A handful of walnuts or almonds every day can help, and so can several different fish, like salmon, halibut, and cod.

Omega 3 Fatty Acids: Much like the aforementioned arginine, Omega 3s are present in walnuts and certain kinds of fish, like salmon. These foods can improve sperm count and cardiovascular health, which by extension, can improve your libido. They also have dopamine-producing qualities, which is one of the happy-go-lucky chemicals released by your brain during an orgasm that can also reduce depression.

THE FLAVORS OF FUCKING

∽

Much emphasis is given to the flavor of her sensual serum or the taste of his erotic elixir. Check out these foods and juices that will help improve how you taste for the next time you want to go down on each other.

Cranberry Juice

Unsweetened cranberry juice (i.e. not *Cran-Ras*) is great for vaginal health. The acids in cranberry juice help restore the pH balance in a woman's vagina, which in turn balances out much of the vaginal ecosystem. Cranberry juice is often recommended to prevent urinary tract infections for the same reason.

Yogurt

Many yogurts or fermented milk products have probiotics, which are the healthy kind of bacteria that help maintain the body's good bacteria and ward off the bad. By maintaining the balance of these microorganisms, a woman's body can defend itself from yeast infections and other problems that affect vaginal health. Many popular Greek yogurts include several probiotics, which is an added benefit because Greek yogurt is high in protein and low in fat.

Fruits and Veggies

Fruits and vegetables that have high amounts of good, natural sugars can help sweeten up his juices. Semen contains natural minerals, like zinc, phosphorus, magnesium, and potassium, which can sometimes give it a metallic taste. Natural sugars from pineapples, apples, lemons, peppermint, oranges, and cinnamon can all help offset this quality.

Good Things that Make You Taste Bad

There are several foods that are super healthy for you but can make your flavor a little rank if you have too much of them, like garlic, asparagus, onions, and broccoli. Raw garlic is incredibly good for your heart (and therefore sex life), but if you're shoveling down a dozen cloves at a time, your juices are going to taste on the poor side. The key to eating these healthy foods without it completely offsetting how you smell and taste is finding an even balance.

BAD THINGS THAT MAKE YOU TASTE BAD

A general rule to keep in mind is that if it's bad for the rest of you, it's probably not doing your flavor any favors either. Excessive alcohol intake, cigarettes, vitamin deficiency, fast food and foods high in saturated and trans fats all make you taste bad. Period.

RESOURCES

Suggested Reading/Watching:

Kerner, Ian, Ph.D., *She Comes First: The Thinking Man's Guide to Pleasuring a Woman*, Regan Books, 2004.

Roach, Mary. *Bonk: The Curious Coupling of Science and Sex,* W.W. Norton & Company, 2009.

The Discovery Channel: Why is Sex Fun? "Volume 3: Why is Sex Fun?". *Curiosity*, The Discovery Channel.

Classy Porn:

X-Art: Classy Erotica, x-art.com

The New Sensations Romance Series, theromanceseries.com

Erotica:

Ravenous Romance Stories:

Dellerman, Jennifer. *Hot Licks*, Ravenous Romance, 2012

Johnson, Cat. *A Cowboy for Christmas*, Ravenous Romance, 2011

You can find plenty more where that came from: visit www.ravenousromance.com for more hot, "inspirational" reads!

OTHER SMUT BY MARISA BENNETT

Fifty Shades of Ecstasy: Fifty Secret Sex Positions for Mind-Blowing Orgasms

From the author of the bestselling *Fifty Shades of Pleasure: A Bedside Companion* comes this naughty new collection of mind-blowing moves! Whether you are single and ready to (co)mingle or married and want to put some new moves into your old routine, pick up this hot how-to and kick your sexcapades up to the next level with fifty new ways to get it on.

If the latest wave of popular erotic romance has gotten your motor running, this book will shift you into high gear!

Author Marisa Bennett steps up again to give you the dirty details on doing the horizontal hula, with wit, humor, and some hot new moves. This guide will help you expand your sexual repertoire and hone your sexytime skills while exploring ecstasy in fifty (count 'em, fifty!) different ways. You'll learn a ton of fun and sexy positions like the visually stimulating Pin-Up Girl, the cozy Lock and Key, and the hot and creative Bobsled (also known as "sledding on Bob"), each one beautifully illustrated to help make sure you've got everything in the proper place.

So what are you waiting for?

Fifty Shades of Pleasure: A Bedside Companion: Sex Secrets that Hurt So Good

Surrender to Your Desire for Naughty Bedroom Pleasures . . .

If hot erotic romance novels have had you fantasizing about certain naughty pleasures, or if you just want to add a little spice to your sexy love sessions, this kinky how-to will bring your fantasies to life. Explore the pleasure of a little pain, flex muscles you didn't know you had through hot sex positions, and learn how to make or break the rules in your playtime romp.

With a light, playful tone, this book eases you into the stingingly sweet side of sex. Each section features excerpts from the Kama Sutra or classic erotica, extra tips like "Dirty Talk Dos and Don'ts," and offers further resources to continue your naughty education. Gather your ben wa balls and feather ticklers while this handbook gives you the rundown on all the hot moves you've been wanting to try, from beginner bondage techniques and starter spanking to hot wax and flogging—no dungeon required!

About the Author

Marisa Bennett is a romance novel aficionado with an English degree and a definite kinky side! She is the author of the bestselling *Fifty Shades of Pleasure: A Bedside Companion,* and *Fifty Shades of Ecstasy: Fifty Secret Sex Positions for Mind-Blowing Orgasms,* as well as some embarrassing fan fiction that may or may not be floating around the Internet.

Her hard limits include ice cream with nuts and skydiving. She now lives with her husband in Minnesota.